M000119126

the little book of
SLEEP

Published by OH!
20 Mortimer Street
London W1T 3JW

Text © 2020 OH!
Design © 2020 OH!

Disclaimer:
This book and the information contained herein are for general
educational and entertainment use only. The contents are not claimed to
be exhaustive, and the book is sold on the understanding that neither the
publishers nor the author are thereby engaged in rendering any kind of
professional services. Users are encouraged to confirm the information
contained herein with other sources and review the information
carefully with their appropriate, qualified service providers. Neither the
publishers nor the author shall have any responsibility to any person
or entity regarding any loss or damage whatsoever, direct or indirect,
consequential, special or exemplary, caused or alleged to be caused, by
the use or misuse of information contained in this book.

All rights reserved. No part of this publication may be reproduced,
stored in a retrieval system, or transmitted in any form or by any means
(including electronic, mechanical, photocopying, recording, or otherwise)
without prior written permission from the publisher.

ISBN 978-1-91161-087-8

Editorial: Lisa Dyer, Victoria Godden
Project manager: Russell Porter
Design: Ben Ruocco
Production: Rachel Burgess

A CIP catalogue record for this book is available from the British Library

Printed in Dubai

10 9 8 7 6 5 4 3 2 1

the little book of
SLEEP

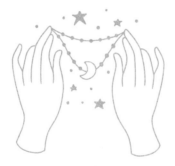

lisa dyer

CONTENTS

Our 24/7 lifestyle is all about being stimulated, entertained and excited; we expect this as an essential part of living and getting the most out of life. Yet, while most of us acknowledge the importance of good nutrition and regular exercise in allowing us to take advantage of our "always-on" culture, we tend to neglect the other essential ingredient for maintaining a productive and healthy life – sleep.

Without a good night's rest, the negative effects soon pile up. Not only is poor-quality sleep linked to irritability, mood swings, poor concentration, anxiety

and depression, but also weight gain,
memory loss, cardiovascular disease,
diabetes and reduced immunity to illness.
Insufficient sleep is linked to 7 of the
15 leading causes of death in the USA,
with the National Institutes of Health
estimating that roughly 30% of people
have disrupted sleep and 10% have
daytime impairment due to poor sleep.

The good news is that better sleep,
in both quality and quantity, can
dramatically improve your everyday life,
long-term health and future happiness.

"There is a time for many words,
and there is also a time for sleep."

Homer, *The Odyssey*

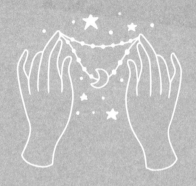

CHAPTER

1

the SLEEP CYCLE

Our lives are governed by a 24-hour internal "clock" called the circadian rhythm, which sets our sleep and wake patterns, ruling everything from hormone production to when we feel like going to bed.

We are all at our most sleepy in the early hours of the morning and again in the early afternoon, which might be why work can seem like such a chore just after lunch.

The circadian rhythm doesn't work alone, however; it also works with light, which is why a streetlight invading your bedroom can make it hard to sleep – *you* might know it's night-time, but your biology can't tell the difference between electricity and the sun.

Our internal clock starts gently telling our body, a few hours before bed, that sleep is approaching by releasing the hormone melatonin. In the morning, our internal clock prepares us for the new day by releasing the stress hormone cortisol into the bloodstream.

the SLEEP CYCLE

Sleep has two main states –
REM (Rapid Eye Movement)
and non-REM. Non-REM sleep
has four stages that take you
into your first hour of your
sleep cycle.

stage one is about 10 minutes long and comprises light sleep. The muscles relax and the brainwave patterns begin to slow down.

During this stage you are very easy to wake, and as it begins, you may have that sensation of "nodding off", with little rouses into consciousness.

stage two lasts 10–15 minutes and you are still in the "entering" stage of sleep, but it would take a louder noise or firmer prod to rouse you.

stage three is a deep sleep in which your brainwaves slow and your heart rate and blood pressure fall. Your breathing becomes slow and regular.

You will need a ringing phone, shouting or shaking to bring you back to the waking world, which would find you groggy and disorientated and probably not very happy!

stage four is even deeper. Your muscles are now totally relaxed and you are difficult to wake up – an onlooker might be tempted to use the phrase "dead to the world".

It is during the deep stage that your body carries out its repair work and fights any illness or damage.

This is the sleep that truly refreshes us.

LIGHT SLEEP

Occurring during stages 1 and 2 of non-REM sleep, this is a transitional sleep, shallower and less restful than deep sleep. It is important for processing memories and emotions and regulating metabolism and takes up 50–60% of your total night's sleep.

DEEP SLEEP

Occurring during stages 3 and 4 of non-REM sleep, this is also called "slow wave" or delta sleep. The more of this you get, the more refreshed you will feel. If you wake up feeling exhausted, you probably did not get enough deep sleep.

This sleep focuses on the physical body to restore energy, regenerate cells, increase blood supply to muscles, promote the growth and repair of bones and tissues and boost the immune system.

did you know? In deep sleep the pituitary gland secretes the human growth hormone.

REM SLEEP

REM sleep begins after the first hour and makes up 20–25% of your night's sleep. Your brain has now started to create some alpha and beta waves, which are similar to the ones produced when awake. You are probably dreaming and your eyeballs are moving under their lids.

Although dreams seem very real, your body won't act out your dreams, as your muscles are paralyzed and you remain motionless. Sleepwalking is likely to happen in the non-REM part of your sleep, which isn't accompanied by paralysis. As the night wears on, the REM stages lengthen and deep sleep becomes shorter.

A full cycle of non-REM and REM sleep takes about 90 minutes: 60 minutes in non-REM sleep, and 10–30 minutes of REM, with the REM sleep periods lengthening gradually through the night. Then the cycle repeats.

The number of cycles you perform depends on how long you sleep, but most people wake up in the final cycle of REM sleep, which is why we often remember our dreams. As you are naturally closer to the waking state at this time, you will feel more refreshed emerging from this sleep stage.

*Even though we may
have slept soundly all
night, we wake up
six times a night on
average – we just don't
remember doing it.*

WHAT HAPPENS WHEN WE SLEEP?

Electroencephalogram (EEG) results show that the parts of the brain that deal with emotional issues are very active during sleep, leading scientists to believe that one of the functions of sleep is to process our daily feelings and consolidate our memories.

Some scientists say we only dream the memories and situations that are meaningful to us, while others consider dreaming to be a way of shedding information that is surplus to requirements.

Humans spend one
third of their life asleep.
They are also the only
mammals to willingly
delay sleep.

LARKS AND OWLS

We are all either "larks" (early birds), which means we prefer to rise early and go to bed early, or "owls", which makes us prone to late nights and later rising times. Larks are often breezy and perky in the morning, but fade fast in the evening. Owls, on the other hand, will loathe an early morning start but find that they are full of energy at night.

Your lifestyle pattern may force you into a set regime, such as taking children to school or shift work, but your natural genetic disposition will decide whether or not you will be at your best when you wake up.

Benjamin Franklin may have said "Early to bed and early to rise, makes a man healthy, wealthy, and wise", however among the highest achieving "owls" are such figures as Winston Churchill, Charles Darwin, James Joyce, Barack Obama and Mark Zuckerberg.

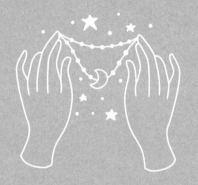

CHAPTER

2

ARE YOU GETTING ENOUGH SLEEP?

The amount of sleep we need varies depending on our age.

Six-month-old babies sleep for up to 16 hours a day; teenagers need about 9 hours; adults need 8; and from middle age the length and quality of sleep often gradually decreases.

Older people generally have greater instances of night-time awakenings, insomnia and unwanted early rising.

Most healthcare professionals recommend 7–9 hours per night, although older people may need less sleep.

You can figure out how much sleep you need by allowing your body to sleep as much as it needs over the course of a few days and logging the hours. You'll then naturally get into your body's best sleep rhythm, which you can continue.

did you know? A giraffe only needs 1.9 hours of sleep a day, whereas a koala averages 22 hours a day.

YOUR SLEEP DEBT

Everyone's needs vary, but research carried out at Stanford University, California, showed that most people had a sleep deficit – or "sleep debt" – of around 25–30 hours at any one time.

Once people had recovered from their sleep debt, they generally settled into a natural pattern of around 8 hours.

If you feel perky in the morning, a little sluggish after lunch and then more alert in the evening, you are getting your sleep balance right.

However, if you dread the sound of the alarm and spend the following morning in a daze, tetchy and distressed, or suffer from frequent colds and viruses, you are probably sleep-deprived.

On average, falling asleep takes 10–15 minutes. If you are falling asleep as soon as your head hits the pillow, it is likely you are not getting enough sleep.

CAN YOU CATCH UP ON SLEEP?

According to one study, it takes four days to fully recover from just one hour of lost sleep. If you try to sleep in on weekend mornings to make up for lost sleep during the week, you may have problems getting to sleep on Sunday night – meaning your deficit carries over to the next week.

If you do plan to catch up on the weekend, sleep for only a maximum of two more hours than you would normally.

signs of SLEEP DEPRIVATION

Excessive sleep deprivation has quite radical effects on the body and studies link it to increased rates of mortality.

did you know? According to Johns Hopkins sleep researcher Patrick Finan, sleep deprivation can age your brain 3–5 years and increase the risk of dementia by 33%.

More than just making you tired, sleep deprivation drains your mental and physical health. Signs include:

- Drowsiness

- Increased appetite

- Inability to concentrate

- Impaired memory

- Reduced physical strength

- Skin conditions, such as eczema and acne

- Increased pain sensitivity

- Mood swings

- Poor balance and coordination

- Disturbed breathing patterns

- Increased risk of accidents

NAPPING

A well-timed 10–20-minute nap can improve your state of mind and your energy levels and help correct your sleep debt.

In many cultures, napping is an accepted and promoted way of living, the Spanish siesta being a prime example.

However, avoid napping if you have chronic sleeping problems, as even a short nap can make it harder to get to sleep at night.

Salvador Dalí took micro-naps he called "Slumber with a Key" that lasted no longer than a second. He would sit in a chair with a heavy metal key pressed between his thumb and forefinger. The moment he fell asleep, the key would fall from his fingers and awaken him.

BENEFITS
of BETTER
SLEEP

Sleep has many benefits,
here are some of the most
important ones:

lifts energy levels: Quality sleep can increase adenosine triphosphate, the energy-carrying molecules in your cells, which surges in the initial hours of sleep.

boosts your immunity to illness: Sleep supports the release of cytokines in your body, the proteins that detect and destroy any foreign invaders your body might be exposed to, such as a virus or cold.

keeps your heart healthy:
Studies found that people who don't get enough sleep are at far greater risk of heart disease or stroke than those who sleep 7–8 hours per night.

improves learning and memory: Sleep allows your brain to organize and process the information that you've taken in during the day and to convert your short-term memories into long-term ones.

helps maintain a healthy weight: Short sleep duration is associated with an increased risk of weight gain in children and adults and poor sleep affects the hormones that signal hunger and fullness.

regulates blood sugar: Studies show that blood sugar levels are disrupted after as little as a week of insufficient sleep.

stabilizes mood: A lack of sleep can make you more agitated and short-tempered, while a good night's sleep improves your ability to stay calm, cool and collected.

reduces stress levels: Sleep allows your mind to unwind and de-stress while insufficient sleep can lead increased cortisol, the stress hormone.

*"A good laugh and
a long sleep are the
best cures in the
doctor's book."*

IRISH PROVERB

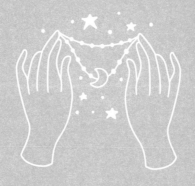

CHAPTER
3

SLEEP
PROBLEMS
and
SOLUTIONS

"*Insomnia
is a glamorous term
for thoughts you
forgot to have in
the day.*"

ALAIN DE BOTTON

TYPES
of INSOMNIA

Insomnia is a catch-all term used to describe a wide variety of symptoms with varying degrees of severity.

primary insomnia is classified as disturbance to sleep lasting at least a month with no obvious physical or medical cause.

secondary insomnia is a side effect of a separate complaint, such as asthma or depression.

Causes can be **intrinsic** (within the body, such as sleep apnoea) or **extrinsic** (alcohol-disturbed sleep, a noisy sleeping environment or emotional distress).

Knowing your particular problem and its cause will help you find the best way to manage it.

SLEEP STATE MISPERCEPTION:

When you believe you have slept much less than you actually have, this can leave you feeling distressed and anxious, even though you have had adequate sleep.

ADVANCED SLEEP PHASE SYNDROME:

Characterized by going to bed too early – and subsequently being wide awake at 2am!

DELAYED SLEEP PHASE SYNDROME:

The inability to fall asleep within two hours of the desired sleep time, usually lying in bed worrying about how you will get up in the morning for work.

PARASOMNIA:

Disrupted sleeping where you may fall asleep easily only to wake fitfully as the night goes on.

This can include the separate conditions of teeth grinding (bruxism), night terrors, sleeptalking and somnambulism (movement while asleep, including sleepwalking).

TRICKS for GETTING BACK to SLEEP

don't toss and turn

This can work you up into even
more of an agitated state.

try progressive relaxation

Working upward from your feet, tense
and release every muscle in your body
while breathing slowly and deeply.
Repeat for as long as you need to.

do guided visualization

Imagine you are in a calm and soothing
place, such as a beach, forest or your
favourite place in the world. Focus on
the sights and sounds you see.

count backwards Slowly count from 100 to ease an overactive mind.

get up! If you can't sleep after 20 minutes, get up. Catch up on boring tasks such as ironing or washing up, or listen to quiet music or an audio book. Avoid re-stimulating your brain by going online or watching television.

resist the urge to watch the clock This can make you more stressed that you aren't getting enough sleep. Turn the clockface to the wall or put your watch or phone in a drawer.

27% of people believe that sleep is more important to wellness than eating a balanced diet and exercising 30 minutes a day, but they still leave it at the bottom of their priorities.

SNORING

Snoring affects around 3.5 million people in Britain, according to the British Snoring and Sleep Apnoea Association, and it is mostly men who snore. It can be caused by being overweight as well as by nasal congestion. The good news is that 99% of snoring cases can be treated.

SOLUTIONS:

Nasal strips can improve airflow.

Drink less alcohol, exercise more and reduce your weight if you are overweight.

did you know? The world's loudest snore is 111.6 decibels – that's as loud as a jet plane!

SLEEP APNOEA

Sufferers may stop breathing for 10–25 seconds at a time. This depletes the bloodstream and deprives the brain of vital oxygen supplies, which makes it suddenly send out an emergency signal, telling the person to wake up and take in a big gulp of air. Sufferers may experience up to 350 "apnoeic events" a night.

SOLUTION:

A continuous positive airway pressure (CPAP) device can ensure you get the oxygen you need.

RESTLESS LEG SYNDROME

Mainly associated with old age, RLS causes a tingling, itching sensation and unexplained aches and pains in the lower limbs. Sleep is disturbed because people have a strong urge to move the legs to relieve the discomfort.

SOLUTIONS:

Massaging the legs, using a hot or cold pack, leg stretches, magnesium and iron supplements or a warm bath can all help.

SLEEPWALKING

Accidents, injuries and even violent crimes have been reported during sleepwalking. Occurring during non-REM deep sleep, the sleepwalker is unlikely to be very responsive or coherent during an episode or to remember the event. Causes can be genetic, environmental or stress-related.

SOLUTIONS:

Gently guide a sleepwalker back to bed – an abrupt awakening can make them fearful or confused – and eliminate any safety hazards.

Relaxation techniques and improved sleep hygiene can help.

did you know? The "sleepwalking defence"– that the suspect isn't liable for murder because they committed the crime without consciousness or intent while sleepwalking — has been argued in courts since the 1870s.

NARCOLEPSY

A condition where you fall asleep at random intervals. It can also describe cataplectic attacks, in which a person abruptly collapses but is actually wide awake.

An attack is often brought on by intense emotions, such as anger or sexual arousal. One person in a thousand suffers from this.

DAYTIME SLEEPINESS

Most people experience this as an early afternoon dip, but hypersomnia is long-term excessive daytime tiredness, where sufferers can go into phases of deep sleep lasting up to two hours at a time.

SOLUTIONS:

Avoid eating refined carbohydrates, such as white bread, and opt for slow-releasing energy foods. Keep away from caffeine and alcohol and don't work or socialize late into the evening.

TIRED ALL
THE TIME

Persistent fatigue, even when first awake, and muscle "heaviness" is often caused by long-term poor sleep habits. However, iron deficiency anaemia can be an underlying condition, as can vitamin deficiency, an underactive thyroid and stomach problems.

SOLUTIONS:

Address any possible medical cause. Eat a balanced diet, reduce stress and practice good sleep hygiene.

SEASONAL AFFECTIVE DISORDER (SAD)

As the winter nights draw in, many people find themselves sleeping longer, eating more and generally feeling low and lacking in motivation.

SOLUTIONS:

Light therapy can be used to increase exposure, but you can also try using brighter daylight bulbs in your home.

STRESS

Stress can motivate us to achieve our goals and respond to constantly changing demands; in its worst form it can give us feelings of anxiety, depression, guilt, isolation, back pain, insomnia and headaches. Learning to manage our reaction to stress is essential to achieving a good night's sleep.

SOLUTIONS:

Any relaxation technique can help, while cognitive behaviour therapy (CBT) can address the underlying issues.

ANXIETY

Ranging from a nervous feeling to a full-blown panic attack, anxiety may have a reasonable cause, such as money problems, but "free-floating anxiety" may persist long after the problem is resolved. It may even be that an unpleasant sleep association has developed, making sleep itself a trigger for anxiety.

SOLUTIONS:

Diaphragmatic breathing (see page 147) can help panic attacks and aid relaxation, or try cognitive behavioural therapy.

DEPRESSION

Sleep disorders and depression are frequent bedfellows. Depression can take many forms, such as being unable to fall asleep, waking frequently in the night or incredibly early, or sleeping a disproportionate amount of time. Other symptoms may include a sense of hopelessness, weight loss, withdrawal, fatigue, indecision and lack of focus.

SOLUTION:

Always seek professional advice.

"The best bridge
between despair
and hope is a good
night's sleep."

E. JOSEPH COSSMAN

SLEEP BRUXISM

Clenching or grinding the teeth during sleep is a movement disorder that can be severe enough to result in an aching jaw, damaged teeth and headaches. You are at increased risk if you suffer from stress, are on medication or have other sleep-related disorders.

SOLUTIONS:

Mouthguards can be fitted by your dentist and relaxation techniques can alleviate stress.

SLEEPTALKING

Known as somniloquy, this is a parasomnia that can result in quite loud talking, shouting or mumbling noises during sleep, mostly unintelligible.

When it occurs during REM sleep, it is known as "dream speech" and related to an ongoing dream. It is harmless, but often caused by stress.

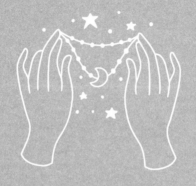

CHAPTER

4

LIFESTYLE, DIET and SLEEP

Whether you are staying up to work, study or have a good time, those late nights may be making you sick.

When the circadian rhythm is thrown off, so is your immune system, which not only can make you more susceptible to viruses, but can trigger inflammatory disorders, such as heart disease, asthma and chronic pain.

*"I'm always on the go.
I love doing things
until I hit rock bottom.
Then I need my
12 hours of sleep, and
I'm on the go again."*

MARIA SHARAPOVA

WORKING AT NIGHT

The very existence of the "darkness" hormone melatonin, which is produced at night to tell us to go to bed, is a clear sign that we are not nocturnal creatures.

People who work shifts for a number of years are more likely to suffer from depression, heart disease and certain cancers, such as breast cancer in women.

stick to the same shift regularly Avoid switching from one set of hours to another.

simulate day and night Make sure the light is bright when you are working and dark when you are sleeping.

power nap Take a 15-minute "power nap" before the start of your shift.

HOW to AVOID JET LAG

The "travel hangover" that comes from skipping time zones can wreak havoc on the body clock and sleep patterns, resulting in disorientation, nausea, headaches and insomnia.

Here are some tips to reduce the effects:

As soon as you get on the flight, set your watch to the new time and act accordingly – if it's 3am at your destination, try to sleep.

Make changes in the week before you fly: get up an hour later/earlier to adjust to the new time.

Don't wake up for the airline meals. Take your own snacks to eat at the right time.

Drink water to help your body deal with the changes and avoid dehydrating tea, coffee and alcohol.

Earplugs, eye masks and the reading light can help you to make your own sun and moon. Use them to control your sense of the time of day.

Take a power nap (no more than 90 minutes) to refresh your brain on arrival, and then get out and about.

THERE'S A NEW BABY IN THE HOUSE

A new baby will almost always have a profound impact on the sleep quality of everyone in the household. Understanding the sleep process and patterns of your growing child can help, but ultimately the best thing to remember is that each phase is just that, a phase.

Here are some sleep survival tips:

- Sleep when your baby sleeps.

- Expose your baby to light and noise during the day to encourage them to sleep more at night.

- Put your baby to bed drowsy but not asleep, as they are more likely to become "self- soothers" and to fall asleep independently.

did you know? A newborn will sleep up to 16 hours a night, a five-year-old needs about 11 hours a night and a nine-year-old roughly 10 hours.

WAKING A SLEEPING BABY

Don't worry about waking your sleeping baby. Track how much time your baby is spending asleep and wake them if they are sleeping too long – oversleeping can mean that they will have more difficulty getting to sleep the next time.

Neuroscientists have concluded that babies don't dream in the same way as older children and adults – it isn't until the age of seven or eight when children experience their first memorable dreams.

BOOSTING BRAIN POWER

Sleep is especially vital for young adults still at school or university, as it promotes concentration, memory and analytical thought, and consolidates learning.

It also has profound effects on their mental and emotional states, physical wellbeing and social development.

Up to 60% of all university students suffer from a poor sleep quality and 8% meet all the criteria of an insomnia disorder.

SLEEP WELL TO LOSE WEIGHT

Research has found that sleeping less than the recommended amount is linked to greater body fat, increased risk of obesity and can also affect how easily you lose weight on a calorie-controlled diet.

Reduced sleep decreases the hormone leptin, which is responsible for reducing appetite, while increasing ghrelin, which increases appetite.

EXERCISE DURING THE DAY

According to a study by the Johns Hopkins Center for Sleep, moderate aerobic exercise increases the amount of deep sleep you get and helps you to fall asleep more quickly.

Exercise helps stabilize your mood and decompress the mind, both important for transitioning to sleep.

However, finish exercising at least three hours before bed.

LIMIT YOUR CAFFEINE

The most widely used drug in the world, caffeine will keep you awake well into the night if you let it, so enjoy your last cup at least five hours before bedtime.

Caffeine is also found in chocolate, cocoa, some energy drinks and even cold and headache remedies and painkillers, so make sure you don't end up reaching for it in other forms.

STOP SMOKING

According to a study by Florida Atlantic University and Harvard Medical School, nicotine intake during the evening, whether through vaping or a regular cigarette, was even more strongly associated with disrupted sleep than caffeine, and resulted in a 43-minute reduction in sleep duration on average.

AVOID ALCOHOL

As a sedative, alcohol helps you *fall* to sleep by making you feel drowsy, but it then proceeds to ruin the rest of your night. Even a small amount of alcohol can reduce REM sleep as well as the length of sleep, with more awakenings and shallow sleep.

It also makes sleep conditions such as apnoea and snoring more pronounced.

REDUCE SUGAR

People who have a diet high in sugar tend to sleep less deeply and have more restless sleep, according to a study by the National Institutes of Health.

Blood sugar levels can crash after consuming sugar, leaving you even more tired and hunting around for another snack to give you a quick energy fix, contributing to an unhealthy cycle.

TRY TRYPTOPHAN

For all the food and drink that overstimulates us and keeps us awake at night, nature has provided us with a sleep-inducing alternative.

Tryptophan is an amino acid that has the effect of speeding up the onset of sleep, decreasing the number of spontaneous awakenings and increasing the overall length of sleep.

Foods rich in tryptophan:

- **Bananas**
- **Turkey**
- **Milk and other dairy products**
- **Almonds**
- **Cabbage**
- **Kidney or lima beans**
- **Oats**
- **Poppy seeds**
- **Pumpkin seeds**

- Spinach
- Wheat
- Evening primrose seeds
- Poultry
- Eggs
- Red meats
- Soybeans
- Tofu
- Basil
- Dill

SLEEP-INDUCING DRINKS

It's true! The traditional glass of warm milk before bed does indeed have calming properties!

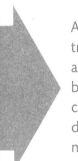

A warm glass of milk contains tryptophan, calcium and magnesium, all of which help the mind and body relax. You can also add a little cinnamon, which is excellent for digestion and can ease an irritating night-time cough.

Herbal tea blends can also be a wonderful way to send you off to sleep. On the following pages are some for you to try.

PASSIONFLOWER

A sedative and digestive aid, passionflower is considered to be a mildly effective treatment for anxiety and insomnia and is often combined with valerian and hops.

It isn't as potent as some of the other natural sedatives, but ideal for those who also get a nervous stomach. Take it in the tea form, three times daily.

CHAMOMILE

As well as in a tea, chamomile can also be used to create a soothing, sleep-inducing bath before bedtime by simply putting a tea bag or two into the bath or floating some of the dried flower heads in the water.

LEMON BALM

This strong lemon-smelling member of the mint family can be made into tea.

Also try using it to season soups, salads, or as a cooling iced tea on hot, restless summer nights.

VERBENA

Also known as lemon verbena, this is similar in flavour to lemon balm, but with a stronger taste, and has similar effects.

LIME FLOWER

Also known as linden, this has soporific effects. Infuse a handful of dried flowers in 1 litre (2¼ pints) of boiling water, and drink two large cups before going to bed.

SLEEP AID SUPPLEMENTS

Some vitamin and mineral supplements can aid sleep. Vitamin B complex should not be taken at night, however, as it can stimulate brain activity.

VITAMIN B COMPLEX

B vitamins help the body cope in times of stress, which is a leading cause of insomnia.

To be most effective, a vitamin B complex must contain thiamine, riboflavin, niacin, folate and B12.

Boost your intake by eating poultry, green leafy vegetables, fish, nuts, seeds, wholegrain products, red meat, soya, potatoes and yeast.

MAGNESIUM

Needed for more than 300 biochemical reactions, magnesium activates the parasympathetic nervous system, keeping you calm and relaxed, and binds to gamma-aminobutyric acid (GABA), the neurotransmitter used in sleep medications.

You will find it in apples, nuts, sesame seeds, figs, lemons and green vegetables.

EVENING PRIMROSE OIL

As well as its high level of tryptophan and gamma-linolenic acid (GLA), which helps balance hormone production, this is a great help to women suffering from sleep problems connected with pre-menstrual syndrome (PMS) or menopause.

MELATONIN

This hormone is released by the pineal gland as the sun sets and makes you feel sleepy and ready for bed. It is not available for purchase in some countries, but it is available in the US.

Taking melatonin as a supplement stimulates sleep when the natural cycle is disturbed, making it particularly effective for jet lag.

KAVA KAVA

Native to the South Pacific, the root of the kava (*Piper methysticum*) is well known for its successful use in the treatment of anxiety, depression, restlessness and insomnia. For sedative effects it should be taken one hour before you want to go to bed.

Kava is available in the USA but restricted in some countries, such as Canada, the UK and Germany.

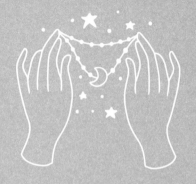

CHAPTER
5

GOOD SLEEP HYGIENE and HABITS

Good "sleep hygiene" refers to the healthy sleep guidelines that improve your ability to fall asleep and stay asleep, as well as the physical environment in which you sleep.

Use these tips to establish a consistent bedtime routine that will optimize your sleep quality. These tips can also be used to re-programme your sleep after an irregular or disrupted period.

1

Make sure you go to bed and wake up at the same time every day, even on weekends.

This helps to programme the body and lets it prepare for the hour when you will want to go to bed.

2

Set a curfew for electronic use – avoid the tv, computer, phone or tablet at least 30 minutes before bedtime.

3

Power down with a consistent pre-sleep bedtime ritual (see Chapter 6).

Try a small tryptophan-rich snack 30 minutes before bed, such as a milky drink, herbal tea, a banana or a few walnuts.

4

Go to sleep when you are truly
tired. If you're not asleep after
20 minutes, get out of bed,
go to another room, and do
something relaxing, like reading
or listening to music until you
are tired enough to sleep.

5

Reserve your bed for sleep.
You want a strong mental
association between your bed
and sleep, so don't be tempted
to hang out in bed with your
computer, work, chatting to
friends or watching TV.

6

Don't sleep in.

Wake up at the same time every day, even if you've had a disrupted night's sleep.

"If you can't sleep,
then get up and
do something instead of
lying there worrying.
It's the worry that
gets you, not the lack
of sleep."

DALE CARNEGIE

If you want to move the time you go to bed – because you are travelling or moving to a different time zone, starting a new job or just resetting your bedtime – do it gradually.

Start at least one week ahead by making small adjustments of 15 minutes at a time.

"Happiness consists of getting enough sleep. Just that, nothing more."

ROBERT A. HEINLEIN

GOOD DAYTIME SLEEP HABITS

Schedule your daytime activities to ensure your body is ready for sleep when night arrives.

1

Follow the sun to support your circadian rhythm. Get a dose of sunshine early in the day and start winding down at sunset.

2

Do your most intense work early in the day when the brain is primed for mental tasks and energy levels are high.

Avoid chores in the evenings – these hours are for relaxation.

3

Limit your caffeine intake – coffee, tea, chocolate or fizzy drinks – to the early part of the day.

Restrict daytime naps to 30 minutes long and take them before 4pm.

4

Regular exercise, especially aerobic activities, promotes deep sleep, but avoid it in the evening, as it will increase your metabolism and overstimulate your brain.

5

Don't eat too late and eat light, avoiding fatty or spicy foods. It can be difficult to fall asleep if your body is still hard at work digesting your dinner.

KEEP A SLEEP DIARY

A daily sleep log will help you to understand if there is a pattern for your poor sleep. For example, do you find yourself unable to sleep the night before important meetings or after working very late?

Sleep diaries often show that although you feel like you may have been awake all night, this is rarely true.

Be sure to track:

- **The time you went to sleep and woke up**

- **Quality of sleep and how you felt the next morning**

- Food and drink
- Medication or drugs
- Exercise
- Emotions and feelings
- Events

did you know? Digital sleep trackers and apps are useful to record the time spent awake, restless and in light, deep and REM sleep. Many also include heart rate and oxygen saturation levels that can raise the alarm on breathing issues.

CHANGE YOUR POSITION

Your sleep position can have an effect on your quality of sleep and your health. If you are a stomach sleeper, your back and neck are at risk of strain. Sleeping on your back exacerbates snoring and sleep apnoea.

Swap to the position recommended by physicians and sleep specialists alike – your side. In this position, the spine remains elongated and relatively neutral.

Dr Chris Idzikowski, director of the Sleep Assessment and Advisory Service, identified six sleeping positions:

the foetal

the log

the yearner

the starfish

the soldier

the freefaller

did you know? 41% of the British population sleep in the foetal position.

CREATING a SLEEP HAVEN

Essential to good sleep is
making sure your bedroom
is an inviting place to sleep –
minimize distractions and mess
and design an environment
that is conducive to rest.

USE QUALITY BEDDING

You move in your sleep up to 60 times in the night, so your bed and mattress needs to give you room to manoeuvre – buy the biggest and best quality you can afford. There are many choices in mattresses, pillows and duvets, so choose the weight and firmness that supports your body and is comfortable.

did you know? After 10 years, a mattress will have deteriorated by as much as 75% from its new condition, so it will need to be replaced.

CHOOSE NATURAL LINENS AND NIGHTWEAR

Linen is kindest on the skin as it is a natural fabric that can help the skin breathe and maintain body temperature. It can absorb up to 20% of its own weight in moisture, thus absorbing the ½ pint of water lost every night in perspiration.

The higher the thread count, the finer the weave and the softer it will feel on the skin.

*Because your body's
temperature decreases
during sleep,
reaching a low point
at daybreak, a
cool room temperature
of 18°C (65°F) is
optimal to sleeping well.*

ADJUST LIGHTING

For the body to activate the "go to sleep" hormone melatonin, it needs darkness. Gentle, low "mood" lighting in the bedroom allows the body to slowly prepare for sleep.

While it is necessary to keep enough light out of the room so you can nod off, you also need to make sure that the there is enough light in the morning to let your body know when to start waking up – so blackout curtains or heavy drapes *aren't* the best choice.

CHOOSE RESTFUL COLOURS

Avoid choosing stimulating colours
such as red, orange and yellow for your
bedroom walls and furnishings; instead
try neutral or reflective colours that most
resemble those found in nature.

REDUCE NOISE

If you live on a busy road, you may need to invest in double glazing, insulation between floors and walls, and ear plugs, or simply move your bedroom to the quietest spot of the house, away from busy main roads.

DISCONNECT ELECTRONICS

Ideally, remove all electronic equipment, such as televisions and phones, from your bedroom entirely, or store them in cupboards where their standby or charging lights can't be seen.

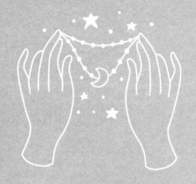

CHAPTER

6

BEDTIME
RITUALS

Practising a consistent
bedtime ritual an hour or
so before your scheduled
bedtime will help you prepare
for a good night's sleep,
unwind the mind and body
and reinforce healthy
sleeping habits.

To make this really effective,
do the routine at the same
time each evening and in the
same order. You deserve to
have a restful night's sleep!

- Read or listen to music quietly

- Dim the lights

- Write down three things that went well that day, and three things that didn't, in your journal

- Make a to-do list for tomorrow, then put it out of the way and out of mind

- Try low-impact stretching or gentle yoga, such as yoga nidra

- Take a relaxing bath with Epsom salts to ease muscles and de-stress

- Practise meditation, visualization or deep breathing exercises

- Treat yourself to self-massage, acupressure or reflexology

- Drink a non-caffeinated beverage, such as warm milk or herbal tea

- Use an essential oil, such as chamomile or lavender, in a diffuser or pillow spray

CREATIVE VISUALIZATION

Imagine you are in a serene place. Notice all the sensations that are associated with this place – the warmth of the sun on your skin, the babbling sound of a mountain stream and even the smell of the grass.

Once relaxed, focus on your breathing. Imagine the stresses and tensions of your muscles as a colour, leaving your body as you breathe out.

BREATHING TO SLEEP

Used in yoga, diaphragmatic, or "belly", breathing is profoundly relaxing. To do this, fully engage your abdominal muscles and breathe through your nose for three seconds, then breathe out through your mouth for three seconds.

Pause for three seconds before repeating. Notice your stomach rising and falling. Practise for 10 minutes each night to wind down.

YOGA NIDRA

A combination of breathing and meditation practised in the corpse pose, yoga nidra balances the nervous system and helps induce a sleep-like state. It is accompanied by a guided meditation, often starting with sensing the physical body, followed by mindful breathing, then noticing your emotions and thoughts and finally reflection.

CORPSE POSE

Also known as *savasana*, this is a neutral resting pose for deep relaxation that lowers the blood pressure and the heart rate, slows breathing and decreases muscle tension.

To do this, lie on your back with your legs straight, arms at your sides and hands resting at either side of your body, palms upwards. Let your feet drop open and close your eyes. Breathe naturally and relax all the muscles of your body. Stay in the pose for a minimum of five minutes, before gently bringing yourself back to awareness.

AROMATHERAPY

Essential oils, especially lavender, clary sage, chamomile, geranium and lemon balm, are known to be effective for aiding a good night's rest.

Use them as an oil in a diffuser or pillow spray, or try the dried herbs in a sleep pillow.

LIGHT A CANDLE

Candles that contain aromatherapy oils will provide a soothing, flickering, melatonin-triggering low light and a calming fragrance.

did you know? In studies from the medical journal *The Lancet*, essential oils have been shown to be as effective as sleeping pills in the elderly.

BLENDING OILS

Try this blend of essential oils to help you drift off to sleep.

10 drops of roman chamomile essential oil

5 drops of clary sage essential oil

5 drops of bergamot essential oil

Blend the oils well in a clean, dark-coloured glass bottle.

Add one to two drops to a tissue and place it inside your pillow to aid you in falling asleep.

If you prefer to make a diffuser blend that you can enjoy during the hour before bedtime, use a ratio of 2 drops of roman chamomile to 1 drop of clary sage to 1 drop of bergamot.

A RELAXING MASSAGE OIL

You can make your own massage oil, but avoid using stimulating essential oils just because they are the only ones you have to hand. This blend will encourage the onset of slumber:

4 drops of lavender essential oil

3 drops of chamomile essential oil

3 drops of clary sage essential oil

Carrier oil, such as olive, sunflower or almond oil – 1 fluid ounce of carrier oil should have only 12–15 drops of essential oil added.

According to the National Institutes of Health, massage reduces fatigue and encourages more time in the restorative deep sleep.

SHOULDER SELF-MASSAGE

Our shoulders often hold the most stress and tension, especially if we spend most of the day hunched over a desk. This massage can be done at any time you notice any tightness in this area.

1 Use the first two fingers of each hand for this massage.

2 Begin by placing the fingers of your right hand in the hollow just inside your left collarbone, at the base of your neck. Press gently and release.

3 Continue this action along the shoulders, towards the shoulder joint.

4 Repeat five times, then change hands and work on the right shoulder.

did you know? There are 3,000 touch receptors in a fingertip, and massage or touch of any kind can help to reduce the heart rate and lower blood pressure.

FOOT MASSAGE

Our feet carry us around all day, yet are often neglected.

Here is a simple foot massage that relaxes the muscles, relieves tension and improves circulation.

1 Use a little foot cream or massage oil as you work.

2 Hold your feet with your thumbs facing inwards towards the sole, and gradually work around, kneading firmly but gently.

3 Rub in small circular motions on the sole, then work on the upper part of the foot.

4 Work up the calf, towards the heart, in gentle, pressing motions.

5 Press the inside back of the ankle (the slight hollow) with the thumb.

ACUPRESSURE POINTS

An effective and ancient relaxation technique in Traditional Chinese Medicine, acupressure is used on various points of the body to clear blockages of energy and promote deep relaxation.

Try one of these simple methods
15 minutes before sleep.

HEGU POINT

Press the web of skin between your
thumb and forefinger for 2–3 minutes
(using the thumb and forefinger of
your other hand). Then swap hands
and repeat.

NEIGUAN POINT

Turn your left hand palm up.
Count three finger widths down
from your wrist.

Apply a steady pressure between the two
tendons here, then massage in a circular
motion for 4–5 seconds. Repeat on your
other wrist.

SHEN MEN POINT

Pinch the fleshy point on your upper ear between your index finger and thumb. Press, then massage in a circular motion for about 1 minute. Repeat on your other ear.

did you know? In one study in the *International Journal of Nursing Studies*, sleep quality improved in patients after five weeks of acupressure treatment on the Shen Men point of the ear and continued for two weeks after.

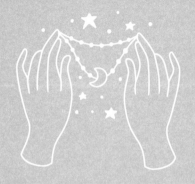

CHAPTER

7

DREAMING

and DREAMS

Dreaming is thought to be a way of processing emotions, thoughts and events from the day. It may act like a "reboot", storing information and memories you need and discarding those you don't.

Dreams are most vividly experienced during REM sleep, and you spend a total of about two hours each night dreaming, often having five episodes of 15–40-minute duration.

More than 80% of
people under 30 dream
in colour, but just over
10% of people dream
entirely in black and
white their whole lives.

REMEMBERING YOUR DREAMS

To hang onto your dreams, remind
yourself that you want to recall your
dreams before you go to sleep.

Don't set an alarm, and do this on a
morning when you won't be rushed.
Wake up very slowly, drifting in and
out of sleep if you can. Play back your
dreams in your mind.

*Within five minutes
of waking up,
50% of your dream
is forgotten.
After an additional
five minutes,
90% of recollection
is gone.*

DREAM JOURNALING

A useful way to capture your dreams is to record them in a dream journal.

Note the colours, scenery and storyline as well as the feelings you experienced and the general emotional landscape. Try to capture as much as you can and note recurring objects, people, places or motifs.

Review your dream journal regularly and look for patterns. Do certain themes or people return again and again? They may help you unlock concerns, relationship issues or stumbling blocks in your daytime life.

*"Dreaming
permits each and every
one of us to be
quietly and safely insane
every night."*

CHARLES FISHER

LUCID DREAMING

A brain state between REM sleep and wakefulness, lucid dreaming occurs when you are aware that you are dreaming.

With practise, some people are able to actively direct their dreams and change the plot or outcome. Lucid dreaming can be used as a tool for self-exploration to reveal your motivations or concerns and reframe them.

DREAM INDUCTION

To make sure you dream at night, use this mnemonic technique.

Before sleeping, write your intention to dream in your journal or on a piece of paper, place it next to your bed, then repeat the intention to yourself over and over again until you fall asleep.

The phrase could be as simple as "I will remember my dreams" or as specific as a dream you want to have about a person or place.

WHY DO WE HAVE NIGHTMARES?

Nightmares can happen any time in life, but usually occur during a period of sleep deprivation or high stress or after experiencing a traumatic event.

Characterized by feelings of distress and accompanied by sweating or a pounding heart, they can wake you suddenly and make it difficult to return to sleep.

If yours are frequent and interfering with your daily life, seek professional help.

"Who's to say that
dreams and nightmares
aren't as real
as the here and now?"

JOHN LENNON

CAN'T SHAKE YOUR NIGHTMARE?

Although fear is the emotion most associated with nightmares, a study at the University of Montreal found that feelings such as confusion, guilt, disgust and sorrow are more likely to stick with you.

IMAGERY REHEARSAL THERAPY (IRT)

Use this technique to counter the negative effects of your bad dreams.

Write down the narrative of your dream, capturing the most frightening aspects, then think about a way to resolve the situation. Give your dream a positive outcome.

Sigmund Freud's
Interpretation of Dreams
regarded dreams as a "royal
road" to the unconscious and
dream analysis as a serious
psychoanalytic technique.

His famous theory was
based on the idea that dreams
represent our repressed
desires and studying them
can unlock our most secret
motivations.

"Dreams are often
most profound
when they seem the
most crazy."

SIGMUND FREUD

COMMON DREAM MEANINGS

Analyzing dream symbols and ascribing meaning to them has become a popular self-help tool to explore your subconscious desires, as well as to reveal concerns and feelings about relationships, work and personal or even global events.

Here are some of the most frequently reported dreams and their associations:

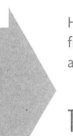

TEETH FALLING OUT

If your teeth are crumbling or falling out, this can indicate a concern with your appearance or a fear of rejection or embarrassment.

It can also relate to communication problems – you literally will find it difficult to speak without your teeth!

BEING CHASED

Are you running away from a particular issue or person?

You are in flight mode and the dream could indicate an inability for you to confront a fear or problem and tackle it head on.

FLYING

Usually considered a very good dream, this can signify that you have set high goals for yourself and you are achieving them.

FALLING

This dream usually signifies a fear of failure or sense of inferiority or being out of control.

You may also need to let go of something to grow and develop.

BEING LATE

This could indicate that you are being deliberately late – you are not sure of the path you are on and so are reluctant to get there.

It could also mean that you are running out of time to accomplish a task or achieve a goal.

FINDING AN UNUSED ROOM

You have new skills you didn't realize you had!

Finding a new room in your home shows you that you are exploring your previously unseen potential.

FINDING YOURSELF NAKED IN PUBLIC

You are in a vulnerable situation and you may be worried your insecurities are about to be revealed.

You may also fear being exposed or wrongly accused.

DEATH

Not a portent of your own death or a loved one's, this usually relates to a fear of the unknown or what your next stage of life might be.

Change may be coming.

"*I dream.
Sometimes I think
that's the only
right thing to do.*"

HARUKI MURAKAMI, *SPUTNIK SWEETHEART*

CONCLUSION

top 10 tips for better sleep

1 Sync with the circadian rhythm and don't fight your "lark" or "owl" tendencies.

2 Go to bed and get up at the same time every day.

3 Don't sleep in, even on weekends.

4 Avoid alcohol and limit your intake of caffeine.

5 Eat a light evening meal.

6 Exercise regularly, but before 7 pm.

7 Practise a relaxing bedtime routine.

8 Create a cool, quiet and comfortable sleep zone.

9 Disconnect electronic devices and any standby lights.

10 Use relaxation techniques to relax your mind and body and induce sleep.

*"A well-spent day
brings happy sleep."*

LEONARDO DA VINCI